Heart   Healthy Delight:

Nourishing Recipes for a Vibrant Life

By:

Alice M.powell

Introduction

Your Guide to Delectable Foods That Are Also Heart-Healthy Introduction

Hello, and thank you for taking the time to visit "Heart-Healthy Delights: Nourishing Recipes for a Vibrant Life"! In this book, we are going to begin on a journey that blends the art of wonderful cooking with the science of eating in a way that is good for your heart. In this article, you will learn the ins and outs of fueling your body, improving your well-being, and appreciating a life that is full of vitality.

Our contemporary ways of living frequently put a huge strain on our hearts. Things like anxiety, inactivity, and the consumption of processed foods all take a toll on the health of our cardiovascular systems. On the other hand, the uplifting news is that we can take ownership of our cardiovascular health and get started on a path toward regeneration just by being more deliberate about the food choices we make.

In this initial part, we would like to welcome you to explore the power of healthy food and its significant influence on both your heart and your entire health and well-being. The science that lies behind a diet that is good for your heart will be investigated, and you will gain an understanding of the essential elements that contribute to optimal cardiovascular function.

As you progress through the book, you will learn how to create delectable dishes without sacrificing the pleasure of eating them or their overall flavor.

Discovering a universe of culinary skills that are geared to optimize nutrition while also tempting your taste senses is something you will do in this course. We hold the belief that eating healthily should never require one to make a compromise but rather be viewed as a celebration of bold tastes and natural, unprocessed products.

We have included throughout this book several recipes that highlight the wide variety of heart-healthy products and cooking options that are available. From energetic breakfasts that get your day off to a good start to satiating salads, nutritious soups, and appealing main dishes, we have painstakingly developed each recipe to give optimal nutrition without compromising flavor or enjoyment. This includes everything from breakfasts that get your day off to a good start to salads, soups, and main courses.

On the other hand, this book is more than simply a collection of recipes; rather, it serves as a guide to help you live a lifestyle that is good for your heart. Alongside each meal, we will provide you with insights and pointers on how to pick ingredients, how to properly limit portions, and how to eat mindfully. Our goal is to equip you with the knowledge you need to make well-informed decisions and adopt a sustainable approach to living a heart-healthy lifestyle.

"Heart-Healthy Delights" is your companion on this fascinating journey, whether your goal is to nurture a vigorous life, manage preexisting illnesses, or prevent heart disease. It is filled with delicious recipes that may help you do any of these things. We encourage you to open yourself up to opportunities, take care of your body, and appreciate the pleasures that are waiting for you on the following pages.

Keep in mind that you are not just looking at a cookbook here. It is a voyage that will refresh your heart, stimulate your body, and get you started on the path to long-term well-being, and it is a transformational experience. These meals are good for your heart and will help you live a life that is full of vitality, joy, and deliciousness. Let the scents, tastes, and brilliant colors of these recipes serve as your guide.

Get ready to start on a journey that will lead to taste while yet being good for your heart. This is the beginning of your adventure, and it is a pleasure for us to be able to serve as your guide along the road.

Chapter 1

The heart secret: Discovering the power of nutritious eating

When we are caught up in the business of our everyday lives, we frequently fail to see the immense power that is contained inside the decisions we make when we sit down to eat. The key to releasing the untapped potential of our hearts and enjoying a life that is rich with energy and well-being is, however, buried deep inside these options themselves. You have arrived at the chapter that reveals the key to a healthy heart: the influence of a diet rich in nutrients.

In this chapter of "Heart-Healthy Delights: Nourishing Recipes for a Vibrant Life," we set out on an adventure of discovery as we investigate the science and magic that lies behind the relationship between food and heart health. We obtain the knowledge and the skills necessary to alter our life and protect the health of our most important organ when we gain an awareness of the enormous influence that the decisions we make about our food may have on our cardiovascular system.

First, we investigate the scientific rationale behind eating a diet that is good for one's heart. We dissect the complex connection between dietary nutrients and the state of one's cardiovascular system using data from the most recent studies as well as the perspectives of leading experts. We shed light on the major players that are responsible for nourishing and fortifying our hearts. These important players include critical vitamins and minerals, heart-protecting antioxidants, and healthy fats.

However, this chapter is not simply a collection of scientific data; rather, it is a celebration of the gastronomic symphony that is in store for you. We would like to extend an invitation to you to start on a voyage through the exciting world of heart-healthy ingredients, where each mouthful is a step towards achieving your utmost potential in terms of health and well-being. We can unleash the real potential of our meals to feed and protect our hearts when we embrace the plethora of healthy foods, fresh vegetables, and nourishing grains that are available to us.

As we progress through the book, you will master the skill of cooking with intention, which involves selecting and preparing products in such a way as to optimize the heart-healthy benefits of those components. We will explore the world of nutritious tastes, fragrant herbs and spices, and the skillful mixing of ingredients that elevate each meal to the level of a culinary masterpiece. Along the way, we will reveal the delectable possibilities that exist inside this universe.

In addition, we investigate the transformational effect of various cooking procedures that improve both the flavor and the nutritional value of the food. We investigate a variety of cooking techniques, ranging from delicate steaming and sautéing to vivid grilling and roasting, to maintain the nutritional value of the ingredients while infusing dishes with delectable tastes.

Not only will you discover recipes in this chapter, but you will also find helpful advice and suggestions on how to adopt a diet that is healthy for your heart into your everyday life. We discuss controlling one's portion sizes, practicing mindful eating, and developing habits that will help one maintain a sustainable and healthy approach to nutrition.

You will not only get knowledge about the foods that protect and feed your heart by using "The Heart's Secret" as your guide, but you will also develop the confidence to experiment, create, and alter recipes to fit your preferences and dietary needs. This is because you will learn about the foods that protect and nourish your heart. Each course is a chance to prioritize the health of your heart while still indulging in the sensual pleasures of dining.

Get ready to discover the heart's secret, acknowledge the power of nourishing eating, and start on a journey that will irrevocably alter your connection to food and the state of your cardiovascular health. Permit the content of these pages to motivate you to begin on a journey toward scrumptiousness and well-being, one in which the heart's secret becomes your most treasured ally in leading a life that is rich in meaning and lively with vitality.

Chapter 2

Rise and shineTo get your day off to a rousing start.

We would like to take this opportunity to welcome you to the section "Heart-Healthy Delights: Nourishing Recipes for a Vibrant Life" which focuses on the power of a healthy breakfast to enliven and refresh your mornings. We are going to go on a gastronomic journey that will reawaken your taste senses while simultaneously supplying your body with the critical nourishment it needs to begin the day on a heart-healthy note.

For a good reason, breakfast has been heralded as the most essential meal of the day for as long as anybody can remember. It gives you the strength and nutrition you need to face whatever challenges the rest of the day brings, therefore setting the tone for the rest of your day. In this chapter, we provide a range of invigorating breakfast recipes that not only titillate your taste sensations but also promote your heart health and general well-being. These recipes are sure to be a welcome addition to your morning routine.

We start by delving into the realm of sunrise smoothies, which are flavorful and nourishing concoctions that are made by blending a variety of fruits, veggies, and superfoods. These effervescent powerhouses provide a revitalizing and energizing beginning to your day since they are loaded with antioxidants, fiber, and necessary vitamins. Each recipe for a smoothie is intended to deliver a nutritious boost while also pleasing your palate. Examples of these recipes include creamy green concoctions and tropical fruit medleys.

As we continue our exploration of breakfast foods, we will now investigate the world of nutritious whole-grain alternatives. These delectable treats for the morning include a range of grains such as oats, quinoa, and whole wheat, which provide you with complex carbs and fiber that will keep you feeling full and energized throughout the day. Each dish is a celebration of the nutritious tastes and textures of the food it creates, from substantial porridges to cozy granola bowls and satisfying pancakes.

In addition to smoothies and grains, we delve into egg dishes that are good for the heart and provide a protein-rich start to the day. Eggs provide a source of complete protein along with critical nutrients such as choline and omega-3 fatty acids, which promote heart health and brain function. Whether you enjoy your eggs scrambled, poached, or in a delightful omelet, eggs are an excellent source of these nutrients.

Throughout the entirety of this chapter, we will stress the significance of maintaining a healthy balance and eating with awareness. We provide pointers on controlling portion sizes, the art of blending components to get maximum nutrition, and strategies to tailor dishes to fit your preferred flavor profile and the requirements of your diet. We think that eating breakfast ought to be a joyful experience that provides nourishment for both the body and the spirit.

Therefore, get up and get going with the assurance that a breakfast that is good for your heart is waiting for you. Allow the intriguing flavors of healthy meals, the brilliant colors of seasonal fruits, and the fragrances of freshly brewed coffee to reawaken your senses and prepare you for an exciting day ahead.

Discover how a heart-healthy breakfast can be a delightful celebration of tastes, textures, and nutrients with "Rise and Shine: Energizing Breakfasts to Kickstart Your Day" as your guide. This book will show you how a heart-healthy breakfast can be. You will find that each dish in this chapter has been meticulously developed to give a mix of critical vitamins and minerals, as well as macronutrients, which will ensure that you get the nourishment you require to flourish.

Therefore, regardless matter whether you're searching for a fast and easy smoothie to drink on the move, a bowl of warm whole grains to savor, or a protein-packed egg dish to fulfill your morning needs, this chapter offers something for everyone. Recognize the importance of starting your day off right by eating a heart-healthy breakfast, and use this meal to lay the groundwork for a day that is full of vitality and satisfaction.

Chapter 3

Salad that sings:Salads that Are Both Refreshing and Satisfying

Salads are a symphony of fresh ingredients, brilliant colors, and enticing aromas that stimulate your palette and feed your body. Welcome to the chapter of "Heart-Healthy Delights: Nourishing Recipes for a Vibrant Life" which celebrates the vibrant world of salads. In this chapter, we will discuss the art of making salads that are not only delicious but also give a fulfilling and heart-healthy start to your meals. Not only will your taste buds thank you, but so will your heart.

The concept of salads as merely side dishes or food for dieting purposes is a thing of the past. They have developed into gastronomic masterpieces that exhibit the elegance and adaptability of fresh vegetables, grains, legumes, and proteins as their primary ingredients. In this section, we will walk you through the process of making salads that are not only beautiful to look at but also include a wealth of beneficial ingredients.

Let's begin by delving into the fascinating world of color pallet salads, which feature a scrumptious selection of colorful veggies and tangy sauces designed to reawaken your taste senses while also providing a wide variety of nutrients. Each component, from tender leafy greens to crunchy veggies, contributes a taste and a feeling all its own, resulting in a congruent synthesis of a variety of flavors and experiences. In this lesson, we are going to investigate a variety of salad dressings that provide a flavorful punch while maintaining a manageable calorie count.

Going forward, we see the potential of grains and legumes to transform our salads into scrumptious and wholesome meals and we embrace this potential. To give our salads more texture, fiber, and a wide variety of important nutrients, we may use sturdy whole grains like quinoa, bulgur, or brown rice. In addition, we go into the realm of legumes, which include chickpeas, lentils, and black beans, all of which pack a powerful protein punch and make our salads more substantial and satiating.

As we move further with our exploration of salads, we will delve into the world of chilled soup sensations, which are revitalizing bowls of deliciousness that blur the boundary between soup and salad. These ingenious inventions blend the greatest aspects of both worlds, making for a refreshing and light appetizer that is suitable for consumption at any time of the year. Each dish for chilled soup, from gazpacho to cucumber dill soup, packs a flavorful and nutritional punch in its unique way.

Throughout the entirety of this chapter, we are going to stress how important it is to incorporate a wide range of tastes, textures, and nutrients into your salads. We offer advice on how to choose the freshest produce, how to make the most of seasonal items, and how to strike a balance between varying flavor profiles. We want each salad to be an experience in flavor, texture, and combination, and we want you to feel encouraged to try new things as a result.

In addition, we are aware of the significance that dressings and vinaigrettes have in boosting the flavor as well as the nutritional content of your salads. We are going to walk you through the process of making homemade dressings that are low in added sweets and bad fats but yet give a wonderful tanginess or creaminess to the dishes you make.

This chapter will provide you with a fulfilling and substantial supper, a light and refreshing appetizer, and inventive ways to increase the number of veggies in your diet. If you are seeking any of these things, you have come to the right place. Each of the salad recipes included in this chapter has been meticulously crafted to offer an explosion of flavor, an abundance of nutrients, and a scrumptious adventure for your taste senses.

Embrace the world of salads that sing, and make them a consistent part of your journey toward maintaining a healthy heart. These salads provide a delicious beginning to your meals and set the tone for a wholesome and exciting eating experience thanks to the combination of fresh fruit, grains, legumes, and dressings that are included in each of the salads.

These salads will take you to a world of gastronomic pleasure and heart-healthy sustenance with their brilliant colors, alluring textures, and harmonized tastes. Grab your favorite salad bowl, channel your inner master chef, and sit back to enjoy the symphony of flavors that will develop with each mouthful.

Chapter 4

Bowls of comforting soups that are good for the heart and the soul.

It is with great pleasure that I welcome you to the section "Heart-Healthy Delights: Nourishing Recipes for a Vibrant Life" which celebrates the reassuring and nourishing world of soups. Soups are a culinary symphony that calms the spirit, feeds the body, and warms the heart. In this chapter, we will start on a journey of flavor and healing, during which we will explore a range of soups that will not only thrill your taste senses but will also promote your heart health and overall well-being.

A piping hot cup of soup possesses a certain enchantment that cannot be denied. It possesses the ability to soothe, heal, and feed one from the inside out. Because of its capacity to sustainably give both nourishment and warmth, soups have long been considered an integral element of the culinary traditions of a wide variety of civilizations. In this chapter, we dig into the art of producing soups that not only satisfy your appetite but also feed your body and enhance the health of your heart.

The realm of broth-based soups, which are light and tasty concoctions that serve as a canvas for a variety of vegetables, grains, and meats, is our first stop in this tour of the soup world. These soups, ranging from the traditional vegetable broth to the fragrant chicken noodle, provide a healthy basis while at the same time enabling the distinct flavors of the particular components to come through. We will walk you through the process of preparing homemade broths, boosting their depth and richness without sacrificing their integrity as a healthy food choice.

Moving forward, we acknowledge the potency of plant-based soups and highlight the availability of vegetables and legumes that can turn a basic broth into a meal that is robust and satiating. Each dish for plant-based soup, from the vivacious minestrone to the silky roasted tomato bisque, is a celebration of tastes, textures, and the nutritional value of the soup's ingredients. To take these soups from the mundane to the remarkable, we are going to investigate the use of spices and herbs as a means of imparting a sense of depth and complexity.

As we continue on our adventure into the world of soup, we delve into the world of creamy pleasures, which are soups that give a rich and velvety texture while still emphasizing the health of the heart. In this lesson, you will learn how to make velvety soups without using a lot of heavy cream or bad fats, allowing you to indulge without sacrificing your good eating habits. These recipes, which range from velvety soup made with butternut squash to opulent soup made with cauliflower, will both warm your heart and feed your body.

In addition, we embrace the varied tastes of soups from throughout the world, serving up bowls of savory and fragrant concoctions that take your taste buds to other locations. Each dish, from the soothing lentil soup to the spicy Thai curry soup, reflects the rich culinary traditions of a distinct country while also using ingredients and methods that are beneficial to the cardiovascular system.

To ensure that your soups have the highest possible level of nutritional content, you must make use of only fresh, entire ingredients throughout this chapter. We offer advice on how to choose food that is in season, how to strike a flavor balance, and how to make the most of spices and herbs to improve not only the flavor but also the health benefits. We think that soups may be a means to embrace a lifestyle that is good for the heart while also being a celebration of gastronomic inventiveness.

In addition, we acknowledge that soups, regardless of their nutritional worth, possess a curative effect. Not only may soups ease the discomfort in our bodies, but they can also calm our minds and spirits. During difficult times, they offer solace, warmth, and sustenance to the person in need. We strongly suggest that you enjoy the process of making homemade soups, allowing their scents and flavors to permeate your kitchen and bringing a sense of calm and well-being to the activity of cooking.

This chapter provides everything you need, whether you're looking for a dish that's light and refreshing to start the meal, something robust and soothing to eat, or a method to include the curative power of soup into your daily life. Each of the nourishing, flavorful, and comforting soup recipes included in this chapter has been painstakingly developed with utmost attention to detail and care.

Explore the world of soups to calm your nerves, and allow the tastes of these dishes to carry you away to a realm of coziness and health.

Chapter 5

Harmony of Nutritiousness: Unleashing the Power of Grains and Proteins

This chapter of "Heart-Healthy Delights: Nourishing Recipes for a Vibrant Life" celebrates the harmonic marriage of grains and protein, a strong partnership that nourishes your body, supports heart health, and unlocks a world of delectable possibilities. I hope you enjoy this chapter as much as I did writing it. In this chapter, we explore the beauty and flexibility of grains and protein sources, demonstrating meals that feed your body, delight your taste buds, and encourage a lively and healthy existence for you and your family.

A diet that is both balanced and good for the heart should prioritize the consumption of grains and protein. Grains are an excellent source of complex carbs, fiber, and vital nutrients, while protein is an excellent source of the important amino acids that are required for the maintenance, development, and repair of muscle tissue as well as the general function of the body. By bringing together these two dietary powerhouses, we can prepare meals that are not only delicious but also beneficial to our bodies.

We start by delving into the fascinating world of whole grains, those nutritious jewels that enrich the mouthfeel, flavor, and nutritional value of the foods you eat. Each type of grain brings to the table its distinct character and set of health advantages, from the nutty flavor of quinoa to the heartiness of brown rice and the adaptability of farro. We will walk you through the steps of cooking these grains to perfection, ensuring that they are juicy, tasty, and keep their nutritious value even after being cooked to the point of perfection.

As we move on, we will explore the domain of protein sources, including those derived from plants as well as those derived from animals, which supply the fundamental components necessary for a healthy body. We take a look at the extensive variety of protein sources that are accessible to you, ranging from lean fowl and fish to beans, tofu, and tempeh. Each dish highlights the adaptability of these components by illustrating the various scrumptious and beneficial ways in which they may be created using the ingredients.

As we move forward in our journey, we are learning to master the skill of preparing meals that are well-balanced and satiating by combining different types of grains and proteins. Each meal in this chapter is a testimony to the harmonious marriage of these two necessary components. From soothing stews and stir-fries to healthy grain bowls and salads filled with protein, each recipe in this chapter is a testament to the harmonious combination of these two vital components. We will walk you through the process of producing great marinades, dressings, and sauces that enhance the natural flavor of grains and protein while also adding a layer of deliciousness to your dishes.

To get the best possible outcomes for one's cardiovascular health, it is essential to prioritize the consumption of cereals that have not been processed and lean sources of protein. We offer advice on controlling portion sizes, planning meals, and striking a healthy balance between macronutrients so that you may eat meals that are not only delicious but also good for you nutritionally.

In addition, we understand the need of catering to individual tastes and dietary restrictions. Whether you follow a vegetarian, vegan, or omnivorous diet, we offer dishes that cater to your requirements and celebrate the multitude of available alternatives. Whether you follow a vegetarian, vegan, or omnivorous diet. We think that a diet designed to keep your heart healthy ought to be inclusive and flexible, enabling you to customize your meals while still emphasizing nutrition and flavor.

This chapter offers something for everyone, whether you are searching for a dinner that is filling and has a lot of protein, a side dish that is based on grains, or an inventive method to include more nutritious components in your diet. Each dish is a demonstration of the power of grains and protein, highlighting their capacity to fuel your body, maintain the health of your heart, and open up a world of gastronomic possibilities.

Embrace the nourishing harmony of grains and protein, and allow the combination of the two to become the basis of your road toward a healthier heart. These dishes provide you with a dynamic and gratifying eating experience while simultaneously feeding your body from the inside out. They do this by including a balance of sources of protein and grains that are rich in nutrients.

Meals that are energizing, satisfying, and supportive of your overall well-being may be created by allowing the textures, tastes, and nutritional advantages of protein sources and grains to come together in perfect harmony. The moment has come to release the power of grains and protein and set off on a journey toward a lifestyle that is nourishing, flavorful, and good for the heart.

Chapter 6

The Enchantment of Vegetables: Vibrant Colors and Delectable Components

The chapter "Heart-Healthy Delights: Nourishing Recipes for a Vibrant Life" celebrates the enchanting world of vegetables and welcomes you to a collection of dishes that display the kaleidoscope of colors, textures, and flavors that vegetables offer to your plate. Welcome to the chapter "Heart-Healthy Delights: Nourishing Recipes for a Vibrant Life" which celebrates the enchanting world of vegetables. In this chapter, we dig into the art of crafting fantastic sides that not only accompany your meals but also steal the show with their brilliance, flavor, and nutritional goodness. These sides will not only complement your meals but also take the spotlight.

Vegetables are a gift from mother nature that bestow upon us a wealth of vital nutrients, fiber, and antioxidants that are beneficial to our health as a whole and our quality of life in general. In this chapter, we would like to urge you to embark on a gastronomic trip with us that investigates the entrancing properties of vegetables, their ability to adapt to a variety of contexts, and their capacity to turn every dish into an exciting and gratifying experience.

To get things started, let's salute the whole spectrum of hues offered by veggies. Every recipe in this area pays homage to the aesthetic joy that veggies offer to your plate, whether it be golden roasted squash or purple eggplant. From brilliant red peppers to vibrant green broccoli, lively red peppers to purple eggplant. We will walk you through the steps of selecting and preparing vegetables to bring out the most of their aesthetic value. This will ensure that each meal is a treat not just for your taste buds but also for your eyes and your sense of sight.

As we move forward, we are committed to mastering the art of bringing out the full potential of the natural tastes and varied textures of vegetables through a variety of cooking methods. We examine the transforming power of heat by demonstrating how it can bring out the natural sweetness, softness, and complexity of a variety of vegetables using a variety of cooking methods, ranging from roasting to grilling to sautéing to steaming. Each of the recipes in this part is a tribute to the wonderful sides that can be made by combining straightforward cooking methods with the copious produce that nature supplies. These recipes may be found in the "Sides" section of our website.

As we continue our exploration of the wonders of vegetables, we will dig into the realm of imaginative and savory vegetable side dishes that will bring dimension, complexity, and the health benefits of vegetables to your meals. Each dish is a celebration of flavor, highlighting how the correct combination of spices, herbs, and seasonings can elevate veggies from basic accompaniments to the stars of the meal. From herb-infused roasted root vegetables to zesty roasted Brussels sprouts with balsamic glaze, each recipe is a standout example of how the right combination of flavors can transform vegetables into the main attraction of a meal. We will walk you through the steps of choosing flavors that complement one another and achieving a balance between the different textures to produce side dishes that are in tune with the main courses you have chosen.

When it comes to the sides of vegetables, we understand the significance of having a wide variety of options and the capacity to be flexible. We offer recipes that cater to your dietary needs and allow you to discover the huge world of veggies, regardless of whether you follow a vegetarian, vegan, or omnivorous diet. These recipes can be found here. There is a delicious grain-based side dish for every occasion and every palette, as well as a light and refreshing salad for every occasion, and it is a vegetable side dish.

Throughout the entirety of this chapter, we will stress the significance of including a wide variety of veggies in your diet to enjoy the advantages that come from eating them nutritionally. We offer advice on where to get fruit that is in season and fresh, how to store veggies so that they keep their freshness, and how to prepare them in a variety of ways that maintain their nutritional value while improving their tastes.

In addition, we are aware of the potential that vegetable sides have to enliven your meals, give them color, and improve their nutritious worth. They are not an afterthought but rather an essential component of a lifestyle that is good for the heart and full of vitality. In this section, we invite you to try out new tastes, play around with a variety of veggies, and let your imagination go wild as you make mouthwatering side dishes that provide nourishment for both your body and your senses.

Therefore, if you are seeking a vegetable side dish that will dazzle your visitors, an accompaniment that will complement your main course in a gourmet way, or a vivid and healthful addition to your regular meals, this chapter offers something for you. The capacity of vegetables to make every dish into a culinary masterpiece is demonstrated by each dish's unique recipe, which serves as a testimonial to the entrancing characteristics of vegetables.

Embrace the enchantment of vegetables and give prominence to the spotlight they cast with their brilliant colors and enticing aromas. With a

These recipes celebrate the magic that veggies bring into your life by using a range of cooking techniques, creative combinations, and a dash of imagination to provide you with a delicious and wholesome dining experience while honoring the wonder that vegetables bring into your life.

Chapter 7

Treats That Won't Make You Feel Guilty: Tempting Snacks & Appetizers

We would like to welcome you to the section "Heart-Healthy Delights: Nourishing Recipes for a Vibrant Life" which fulfills your appetites with guilt-free snacks and appetizers. This section has a selection of dishes that demonstrate that you may partake in mouthwatering delights while still prioritizing your heart health and general well-being. In this chapter, we will investigate the art of preparing scrumptious snacks and appetizers that not only excite your taste buds but also provide your body with the nutrition it needs via the utilization of healthy foods.

Snacks and appetizers are essential components of our culinary journey since they provide us with several opportunities for moments of enjoyment and fulfillment throughout the day. Traditional snacks and appetizers, on the other hand, frequently include unhealthful foods and excessive calories, both of which can be detrimental to the health of our hearts. In this chapter, we welcome you to explore a new world of mouthwatering goodies – alternatives that are both tasty and healthful, giving you the freedom to indulge in your go-to munchies without feeling guilty or having to make sacrifices.

We start by rethinking some of your all-time favorites, giving them a new spin that's better for you while yet retaining their tempting tastes. From handmade crackers made with whole grains to baked vegetable chips that are crispy on the outside and soft on the inside, each dish in this section demonstrates the inventive ways in which traditionally rich snacks can be transformed into joys that are good for the heart. We will walk you through the process of choosing nutrient-dense ingredients, striking a flavor balance, and employing smart cooking procedures that assure both flavor and nourishment in the final product.

Moving forward, we are going to delve into the world of scrumptious dips and spreads, which is a collection of recipes that will give your snacks and appetizers a burst of flavor while also including healthy components. These recipes demonstrate the variety of plant-based foods, highlighting how they can boost the enjoyment of some of your favorite snacks. From fresh and spicy salsas to creamy hummus variants, these recipes range from simple to complex. To make your experience of snacking even more enjoyable, we will give pointers on taste pairings, ideas for component replacements, and presentation concepts.

As we move further on our adventure, we will investigate the world of delectable morsels that may be eaten in one bite. These will be appetizers that will fuel your body while also making a statement. Each recipe in this part is a celebration of the art of appetizers, blending flavor, appearance, and nutrition in perfect harmony. From bright and refreshing summer rolls to savory stuffed mushrooms, this section is a celebration of the art of appetizers. We will walk you through the steps of making bite-sized miracles that will amaze both your visitors and your taste senses, and we will do so with ease.

In addition, we are aware of the need of maintaining a healthy equilibrium and observing proper portion management when it comes to snacks and appetizers. In this chapter, we will provide you with advice on how to eat mindfully, how much food to serve at a time, and how to make intelligent ingredient replacements so that your snacking habits will complement your efforts to improve your heart health. We think that indulging oneself and receiving adequate nutrition are not mutually exclusive, and if you make intelligent decisions, you will be able to satisfy your sweet tooth without jeopardizing your health.

Throughout the entirety of this chapter, we emphasize the significance of making use of fresh, complete products while cooking snacks and appetizers to not only satiate your needs but also supply you with important nutrients. We provide direction on how to choose products that are high in nutrients, how to include a range of flavors and textures, and how to embrace handmade choices that give you control over the quality of your snacks.

In addition, we are aware that snacking and the consumption of appetizers ought to be a source of pleasure and contentment. They are supposed to be appreciated by themselves as well as by other people. In this chapter, we urge you to embrace the social component of snacking, to experiment with flavors and textures, and to let your creativity show through as you make delights that are guilt-free and bring others together to share in the experience.

Therefore, if you are seeking something to perk you up in the middle of the day, spending a peaceful evening at home, or having a get-together, this chapter offers something for you. All of the recipes in this book are living proof that munching on anything between meals can be a pleasurable experience as well as good for your heart. They also provide you with an enticing selection of sweets that are good for your body and stimulate your senses.

Embrace the world of snacks and appetizers that you can enjoy without feeling guilty, and make indulging in these mouthwatering foods a part of your path toward maintaining a healthy heart. Featuring a harmony of healthful ingredients, unique taste combinations

, and shrewd decisions, these recipes ensure that your experience of snacking will be both enjoyable and nourishing; they are a real treat for your taste senses as well as your overall health.

Chapter 8

Sweet Sensations: Indulge in Heartwarming Desserts

It is my pleasure to welcome you to the section "Heart-Healthy Delights: Nourishing Recipes for a Vibrant Life" that invites you to experience the joy of sweet sensations. This chapter features a collection of heartwarming dessert recipes that demonstrate that you can indulge in decadent treats while still prioritizing your heart health and overall well-being. In this chapter, we will discuss the art of making desserts that not only satiate your want for something sweet but also provide your body with the nutrients it needs via the use of healthful ingredients and taste profiles.

Desserts have a unique place in our hearts since they bring up warm and fuzzy sentiments, as well as celebration and sheer enjoyment. On the other hand, classic sweets are frequently filled to the brim with refined sugars, harmful fats, and empty calories, all of which can have a detrimental effect on our health. In this chapter, we want to reinvent desserts by displaying a range of dishes that are both mouthwatering and good for your heart. This will enable you to experience sweet sensations without having to make any sacrifices.

In the first step of our process, we rethink traditional sweets by giving them a more healthful makeover that preserves their delectable flavor while also increasing the amount of nutrients they contain. Each dish in this part showcases the creative potential of transforming decadent desserts into guilt-free pleasures. From a rich and creamy avocado chocolate mousse to fruity and refreshing sorbets, the recipes in this section range from rich and creamy to fruity and refreshing. We will walk you through the steps of choosing natural sweeteners, combining foods high in nutrients, and finding a balance between the many flavors and textures.

As we go on, we explore the world of baked delicacies, which is a collection of dishes that will both make your heart feel warm and your taste senses sing with delight. These recipes showcase the skill of baking using ingredients that are good for the heart, such as whole grains, nuts, and fruits, and range from cakes made with whole grains that are soft and moist to pastries that are delicate and flaky. You will be able to relish the sweetness without jeopardizing your health objectives if you follow the advice that we offer regarding ingredient replacements, controlling portions, and mindful indulging.

As we continue our adventure into the world of desserts, we delve into the realm of frozen pleasures, which are sweets that are both icy and refreshing, and deliver a blast of taste as well as a sense of fulfillment. Each of the recipes in this part demonstrates the diversity of frozen desserts while using wholesome ingredients. From delicious and creamy frozen yogurt to creative and creamy lovely cream, the recipes range from savory to sweet. We will walk you through the process of producing frozen sensations that will not only help you feel more comfortable but will also provide your body with healthy and beneficial ingredients.

When it comes to indulging in sweets, we understand the need of maintaining a healthy equilibrium and eating in proportion at all times. In this chapter, we offer advice on controlling portion sizes, eating mindfully, and indulging in sweets while maintaining a mindful attitude. We are of the opinion that desserts can be part of a healthy and fulfilling lifestyle, and if you make the proper decisions, you may experience the sweetness of sweets while also supporting your heart health and general well-being.

Throughout the entirety of this chapter, we place an emphasis on the use of natural and unprocessed components in order to concoct sweets that not only satiate your needs but also supply important nutrients. We offer guidance on how to choose fruits that are in season and fully ripe, how to include whole grains and nuts in your diet, and how to make use of more nutritious alternatives to processed sugars and bad fats.

In addition, we are aware that desserts serve as much more than simply a delicious conclusion to a meal; they are also a method of commemorating significant occasions, a form of self-care, and an outlet for expressing love and creative expression. In this chapter, we encourage you to embrace the art of dessert creation, to explore with different flavors and textures, and to allow your imagination run wild as you make warm and comforting delights that bring joy not just to yourself but to people around you as well.

This means that whether you're searching for a reassuring baked dessert, a reviving frozen pleasure, or a sugary treat that won't make you feel guilty, this chapter offers something for you to try. Each dessert dish is evidence that sweet treats can be both luxurious and nourishing. They can provide you with a pleasant assortment of sugary sensations that can fulfill your desires while also supporting a lifestyle that is good for your heart.

Entangle yourself in the realm of comforting sweets, and make these sugary experiences a permanent part of your culinary repertoire.

journey. These recipes will guarantee that your experience with dessert is a wonderful and nutritious celebration of life's sweet moments by providing you with a balance of healthful ingredients, thoughtful indulgence, and a touch of creativity in the preparation of the dish.

Conclusion

Your path towards a heart -healthy lifestyle start right now

Congratulations! You have completed "Heart-Healthy Delights: Nourishing Recipes for a Vibrant Life," a culinary journey that has taken you through the worlds of nutritious and delicious meals meant to feed your body, pleasure your senses, and support your heart health. At this point, you have arrived at the conclusion of your culinary adventure. As you get to the end of this book, we want you to take some time to think about the important life lessons and self-improvement advice you've picked up along the road.

Throughout this whole book, we have discussed the strong relationship that exists between the foods we eat and the health of our hearts. We have also emphasized how important it is to make conscious decisions that put both nutrition and flavor first. From the introductory chapters that built the framework for your heart-healthy journey to the fun chapters filled with nutritious recipes, each page has been dedicated to equipping you with information, inspiration, and practical skills to lead a life that is vibrant and meaningful. From the opening chapters that laid the foundation for your heart-healthy journey to the delicious chapters filled with nourishing recipes, each page has been committed to empowering you.

To start, we decoded the mysteries of healthy eating by gaining a knowledge of how the foods we eat influence not only our cardiovascular health but also our general well-being. You have gained an understanding of the value of consuming whole foods and substances derived from plants, as well as the relevance of include a wide range of nutrients in your diet. You now have the knowledge necessary to take the first step toward adopting a lifestyle that is beneficial to your heart.

As you progressed, you were familiar with nourishing breakfasts that provide a jolt of energy at the beginning of the day and fill the mornings with power and sustenance. You delighted in savoring salads that were both fresh and satisfying, reawakening your taste senses as they embraced the vivacious tastes of seasonal fruit. You relished in nourishing soups that nourished both your heart and your spirit, offering comfort and warmth with each and every mouthful that you consumed.

You have unlocked the potential of nutritious grains and protein to provide your body with fuel and improve your overall health by making you aware of their power. Congratulations! You were awestruck by the magic of vegetables as their brilliant hues and mouthwatering accompaniments turned your dishes into works of culinary art. You indulged in snacks and appetizers without feeling guilty, demonstrating that it is possible to enjoy attractive foods without jeopardizing one's cardiovascular health.

And last but not least, you indulged in some mouthwatering sweets, which not only satiated your desires but also provided your body with the healthful tastes and components it needed to function properly. These delectable delicacies served as a gentle reminder that it is possible for pleasure and nourishment to coexist, and that it is possible to honor your health while still celebrating the important moments in life.

However, the contents of this book are not limited to only a compilation of recipes. It is a call to action—a call to begin on a heart-healthy journey that goes beyond the limitations of its pages. This is a call to action. You are extended a welcome to engage in deliberate decision-making in order to nurture all aspects of your being: body, mind, and spirit. It serves as a reminder that robust health is within your reach, and that every tiny step you take toward a heart-healthy lifestyle is a step towards a better and more meaningful future for yourself and your loved ones.

As you put this book away, keep in mind that your road toward a healthy heart starts right now. Apply the new information that you've learned and the ideas that have inspired you to your day-to-day activities. Allow the recipes and insights to serve as a guide, but don't be afraid to let your intuition and imagination run wild as you modify them to suit your one-of-a-kind preferences in flavor and texture.

Embrace the pleasure of making heart-healthy meals for your loved ones, taste the flavors that nature has to offer, and share the happiness of eating in a way that is good for your heart with those you care about. Celebrate the rich life that is ahead of you, one that is full of vitality, energy, and the satisfaction that comes from knowing that you are nourishing your body and supporting the health of your heart.

Your road toward a healthy heart will be ongoing and always changing. It is a commitment to oneself and to one's overall health and happiness. Therefore, let the information, recipes, and ideas contained in this book to serve as a source of motivation for you as you pursue a life that is full of vitality. You are adopting a heart-healthy lifestyle with every meal you cook, every ingredient you select, and every mouthful you appreciate, which will provide you with nourishment for many years to come as a result of your efforts.

We are grateful that you have decided to travel with us. I pray that the nourishing joys of life, together with good health and happiness, will flood your heart.

that contribute to a life that is full of vitality. Keep in mind that the first step toward a healthy heart is taking this very moment.